I'M ALLERGIC TO SOY

By Walter LaPlante

Gareth Stevens
PUBLISHING

Please visit our website, www.garethstevens.com. For a free color catalog of all our high-quality books, call toll free 1-800-542-2595 or fax 1-877-542-2596.

Library of Congress Cataloging-in-Publication Data

Names: LaPlante, Walter, author.
Title: I'm allergic to soy / Walter LaPlante.
Description: New York : Gareth Stevens Publishing, [2019] | Series: I'm allergic | Includes index.
Identifiers: LCCN 2018020799| ISBN 9781538229071 (library bound) | ISBN 9781538232446 (paperback) | ISBN 9781538232453 (6 pack)
Subjects: LCSH: Food allergy–Juvenile literature.
Classification: LCC RC596 .L38 2019 | DDC 616.97/5–dc23
LC record available at https://lccn.loc.gov/2018020799

Published in 2019 by
Gareth Stevens Publishing
111 East 14th Street, Suite 349
New York, NY 10003

Designer: Laura Bowen
Editor: Kate Mikoley

Photo credits: cover, p. 1 (main) Dan76/Shutterstock.com; cover, p. 1 (edamame) NIPAPORN PANYACHAROEN/Shutterstock.com; p. 5 ANURAK PONGPATIMET/Shutterstock.com; p. 7 nnattalli/Shutterstock.com; p. 9 (soup) Elena Shashkina/Shutterstock.com; p. 9 (edamame) Rattana Rattanawan/Shutterstock.com; p. 9 (soy sauce) sevenke/Shutterstock.com; p. 9 (tofu) Elena Veselova/Shutterstock.com; p. 11 Eakachai Leesin/Shutterstock.com; p. 13 michaeljung/Shutterstock.com; p. 15 Photographee.eu/Shutterstock.com; pp. 17, 21 Monkey Business Images/Shutterstock.com; p. 19 andresr/E+/Getty Images.

Printed in the United States of America

CPSIA compliance information: Batch #CW19GS: For further information contact Gareth Stevens, New York, New York at 1-800-542-2595.

CONTENTS

Boldface words appear in the glossary.

A Common Allergy

Soy is a common allergy among children in the United States. About 0.4 percent of children have an allergy to soy. An allergy is the body's **sensitivity** to things in the surroundings that are usually harmless.

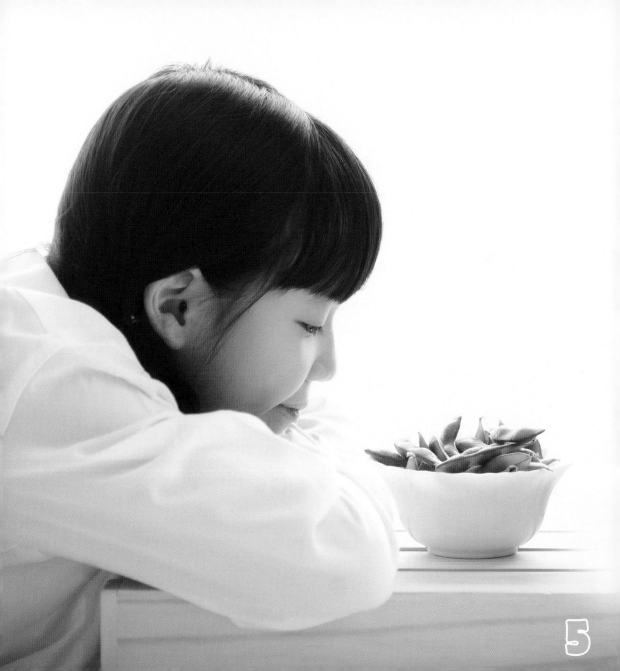

5

Soy comes from the soybean plant. Soybeans are part of the legume family, which also has peas, beans, and peanuts in it. Soybeans can be eaten on their own. They can also be **processed** for use in many kinds of foods.

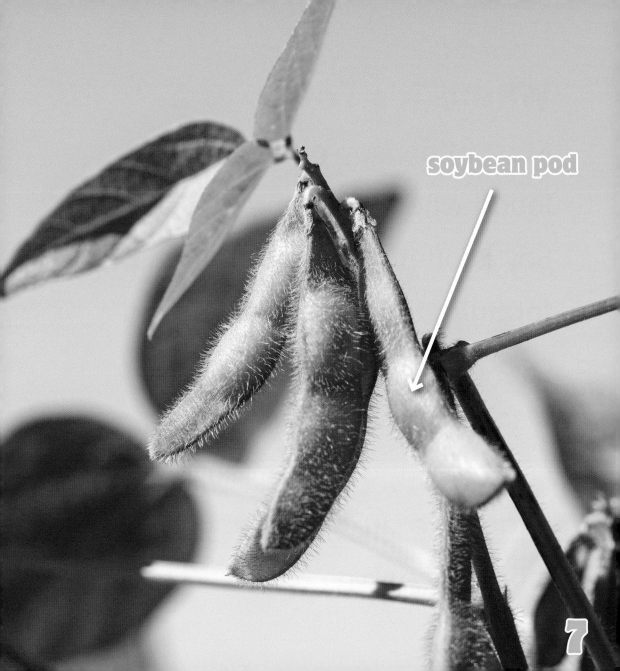

soybean pod

7

Where It's Found

Most often, soy allergies are found when someone is a baby. Soy is often an **ingredient** in baby **formula**. Soy is in some baked goods and canned soups. It's also in soy sauce and tofu, which are made from soybeans. Edamame are young soybeans that are cooked.

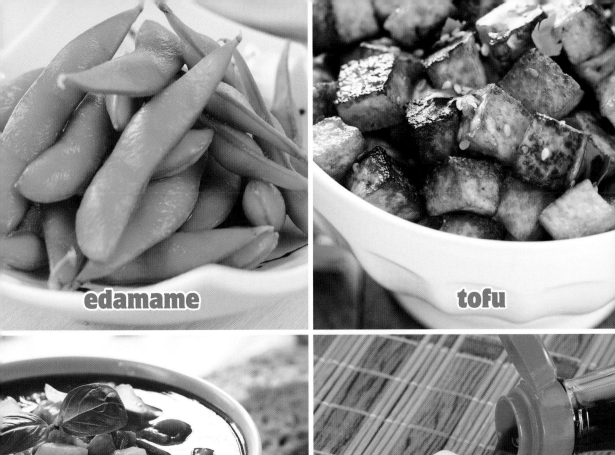
edamame

tofu

soups and baked goods

soy sauce

Sick From Soy

Signs of a soy allergy can happen minutes or hours after eating soy. **Hives**, swelling of part of the face, and **itchiness** are signs of a soy allergy. A runny nose or tummy pain are too. Some people may even throw up!

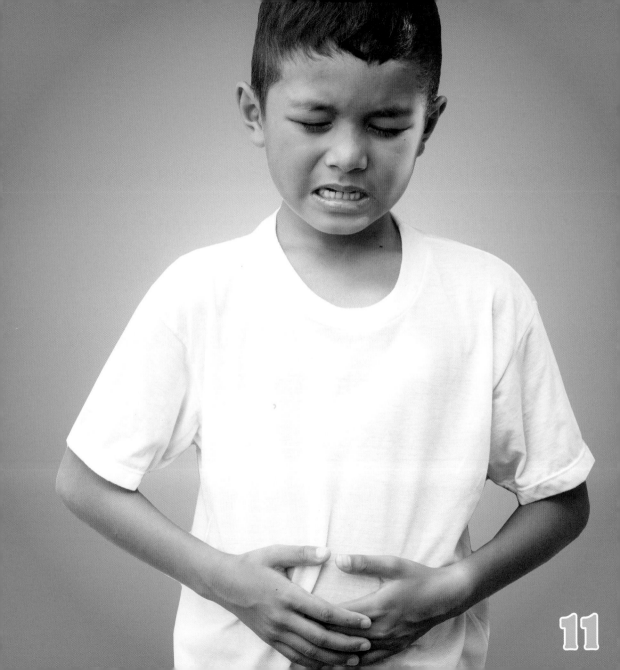

11

Sometimes, someone with a soy allergy may have a serious **reaction**. They can have trouble breathing, feel dizzy, or have a hard time swallowing. This is called anaphylaxis (an-uh-fuh-LAK-sis). They need **medicine** or a doctor's help right away.

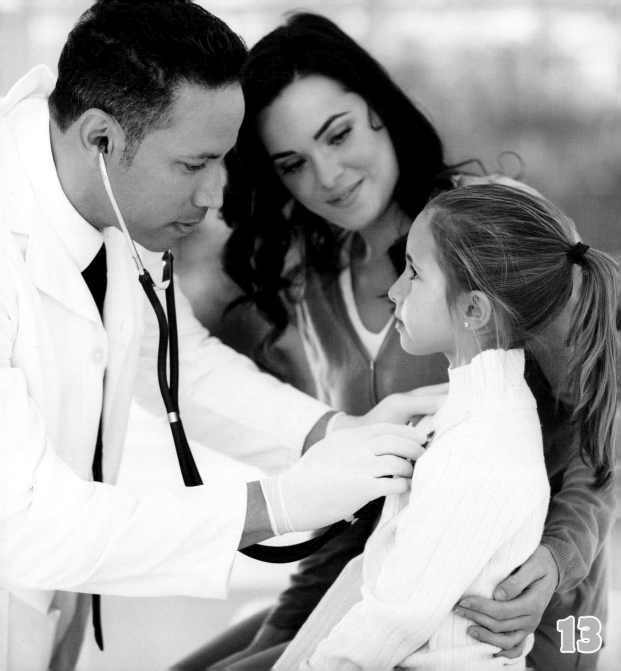

13

Be Sure It's Soy

An allergist, or allergy doctor, can give a blood test to be sure it's soy that's making someone feel sick. The allergist can also **prick** the skin and put soy on it. If the spot gets red and raised, it shows that a person has a soy allergy.

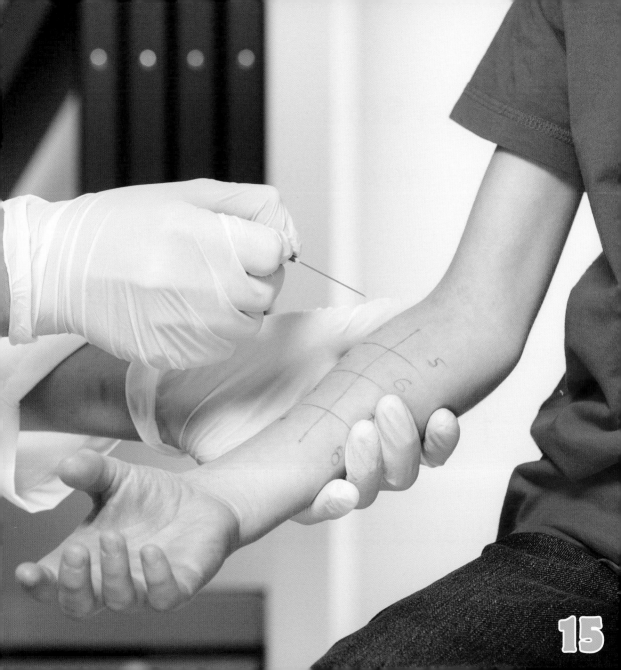

Staying Safe

The best way to take care of a soy allergy is by staying away from food with soy in it! Read the ingredients of foods that come in packages. Many of these foods have an additional label that says there's soy in them.

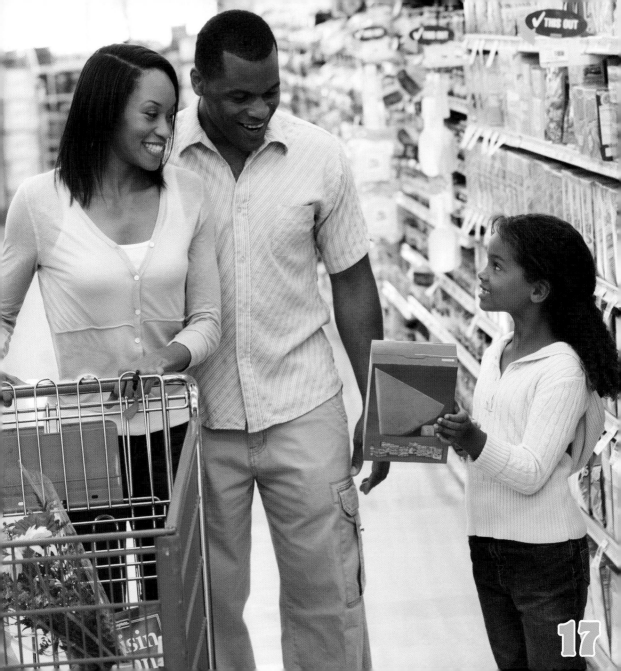

People with soy allergies need to be careful of foods that may have touched soy, too. When eating at a restaurant, let the cook or server know about your allergy. They can help you choose foods that are safe!

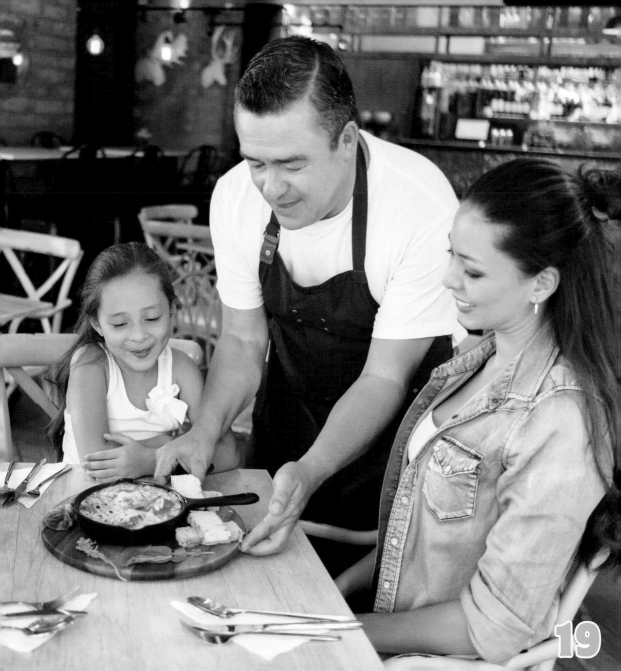

The Good News!

Most children with a soy allergy don't have it their whole life. Many outgrow it by age 10! However, adults have soy allergies, too. No matter your age, staying away from soy is the best way to stop allergic reactions!

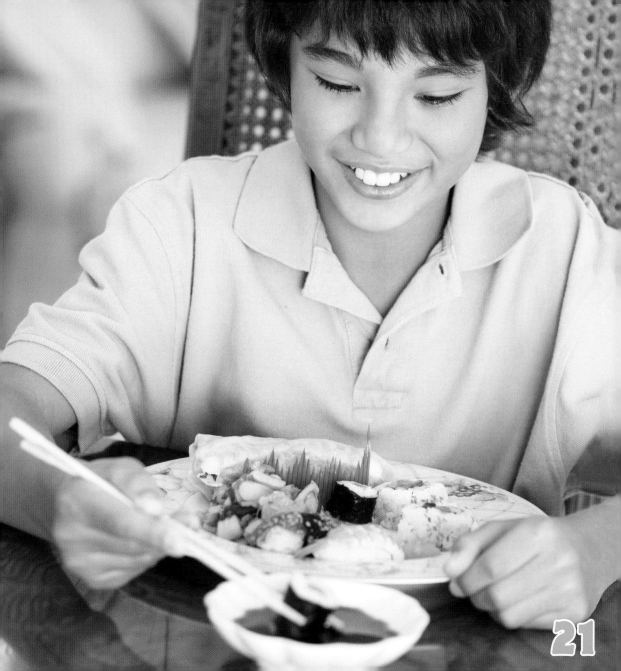

GLOSSARY

formula: a liquid that commonly has milk in it and that is used for feeding a baby

hives: a condition in which part of the skin becomes raised, red, and itchy

ingredient: one of the things used to make food

itchy: having an unpleasant feeling on your skin or inside your mouth or nose that makes you want to scratch

medicine: a drug taken to make a sick person well

prick: to make a very small hole in something

process: to change something from one form into another by preparing, handling, or treating it in a special way

reaction: the way your body acts because of certain matter or surroundings

sensitivity: the state of being easily affected

FOR MORE INFORMATION

BOOKS

Jorgensen, Katrina. *Enjoy Without Soy: Easy and Delicious Soy-Free Recipes for Kids with Allergies.* North Mankato, MN: Capstone Press, 2017.

Potts, Francesca. *All About Allergies.* Minneapolis, MN: Super Sandcastle, 2018.

WEBSITES

Food Allergies
kidshealth.org/en/kids/food-allergies.html
Read all about how the immune system works and why food allergies happen.

Soy Allergy
www.kidswithfoodallergies.org/page/soy-allergy.aspx
Find out how to stay safe when living with a soy allergy.

INDEX